MW00508791

Slow Cooker Breakfast Recipes

Easy, Hands-Off Recipes for Your Slow Cooker

By Paulina Montego

Sommario

Introduction...7

Slow Cooker Breakfast Recipes.........................9

Introduction

We understand you are constantly looking for less complicated means to cook your meals. We likewise recognize you are possibly tired investing long hours in the kitchen food preparation with so many pans as well as pots. Well, currently your search is over! We found the perfect kitchen tool you can utilize from now on! We are discussing the Slow stove! These incredible pots permit you to cook a few of the most effective recipes ever with minimal effort Slow cookers cook your dishes easier and also a great deal healthier! You don't need to be a specialist in the kitchen to cook several of the most scrumptious, flavored, textured and also abundant dishes! All you require is your Slow stove as well as the right components! It will reveal you that you can make some fantastic breakfasts, lunch recipes, side recipes, poultry, meat and fish dishes. Ultimately yet significantly, this cookbook supplies you some simple as well as pleasant desserts.

Slow Cooker Breakfast Recipes

Pork and Cranberries

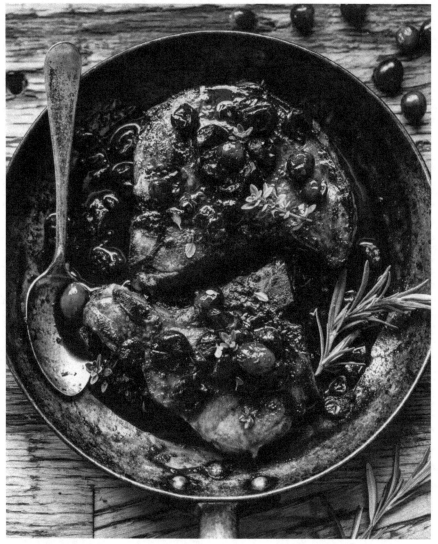

Preparation time: 10 minutes
Cooking time: 8 hours
Servings: 2

Ingredients:

- 1 pound pork tenderloin, roughly cubed
- ½ cup cranberries
- ½ cup red wine
- ½ teaspoon sweet paprika

- ½ teaspoon chili powder
- 1 tablespoon maple syrup

Directions:

1. In your slow cooker, mix the pork with the cranberries, wine and the other ingredients, toss, put the lid on and cook on Low for 8 hours.
2. Divide between plates and serve.

Nutrition: calories 400, fat 12, fiber 8, carbs 18, protein 20

Onion Chicken

Preparation time: 10 minutes
Cooking time: 6 hours
Servings: 2

Ingredients:
- 1 small yellow onion, chopped
- 2 carrots, sliced
- 1 cup green beans
- ½ celery rib, chopped
- 2 chicken breast halves, boneless and skinless
- 2 small red potatoes, halved
- 2 bacon strips, cooked and crumbled
- Salt and black pepper to the taste
- ¾ cup water
- ¼ teaspoon basil, dried
- ¼ teaspoon thyme, dried

Directions:
1. In your Slow cooker, mix onion with carrots, green beans, celery, chicken, red potatoes, bacon, salt, pepper, water, basil and thyme, cover and cook on Low for 6 hours.
2. Divide between plates and serve for lunch.

Nutrition: calories 304, fat 7, fiber 5, carbs 20, protein 37

Lamb and Onion Stew

Preparation time: 10 minutes
Cooking time: 8 hours
Servings: 2

Ingredients:
- 1 pound lamb meat, cubed
- 1 red onion, sliced
- 3 spring onions, sliced
- Salt and black pepper to the taste
- 1 tablespoon olive oil
- ½ teaspoon rosemary, dried
- ¼ teaspoon thyme, dried
- 1 cup water
- ½ cup baby carrots, peeled
- ½ cup tomato sauce
- 1 tablespoon cilantro, chopped

Directions:
1. In your slow cooker, mix the lamb with the onion, spring onions and the other ingredients, toss, put the lid on and cook on Low for 8 hours.
2. Divide the stew between plates and serve hot.

Nutrition: calories 350, fat 8, fiber 3, carbs 14, protein 16

Beef Chili

Preparation time: 10 minutes
Cooking time: 6 hours
Servings: 8

Ingredients:
- 3 chipotle chili peppers in adobo sauce, chopped
- 2 pounds beef steak, cubed
- 1 yellow onion, chopped
- 2 garlic cloves, minced
- 1 tablespoon chili powder
- Salt and black pepper to the taste
- 45 canned tomato puree
- ½ teaspoon cumin, ground
- 14 ounces beef stock
- 2 tablespoons cilantro, chopped

Directions:
1. In your Slow cooker, chipotle chilies with beef, onion, garlic, chili powder, salt, pepper, tomato puree, cumin and stock, stir, cover and cook on Low for 6 hours.
2. Add cilantro, stir, divide into bowls and serve for lunch.

Nutrition: calories 230, fat 8, fiber 2, carbs 12, protein 25

Pork Roast and Olives

Preparation time: 10 minutes
Cooking time: 6 hours
Servings: 2

Ingredients:
- 1 pound pork roast, sliced
- ½ cup black olives, pitted and halved
- ½ cup kalamata olives, pitted and halved
- 2 medium carrots, chopped
- ½ cup tomato sauce
- 1 small yellow onion, chopped
- 2 garlic cloves, minced
- 1 bay leaf
- Salt and black pepper to the taste

Directions:
1. In your slow cooker, mix the pork roast with the olives and the other ingredients, toss, put the lid on and cook on High for 6 hours.
2. Divide everything between plates and serve.

Nutrition: calories 360, fat 4, fiber 3, carbs 17, protein 27

Moist Pork Loin

Preparation time: 10 minutes
Cooking time: 5 hours
Servings: 8

Ingredients:
- 3 pound pork loin roast
- 1 teaspoon onion powder
- 1 teaspoon mustard powder
- 2 cups chicken stock
- 2 tablespoons olive oil
- ¼ cup cornstarch
- ¼ cup water

Directions:
1. In your Slow cooker, mix pork with onion powder, mustard powder, stock and oil, cover and cook on Low for 5 hours.
2. Transfer roast to a cutting board, slice and divide between plates.
3. Transfer cooking juices to a pan and heat it up over medium heat.
4. Add water and cornstarch, stir, cook until it thickens, drizzle over roast and serve for lunch.

Nutrition: calories 300, fat 11, fiber 1, carbs 10, protein 34

Beef Stew

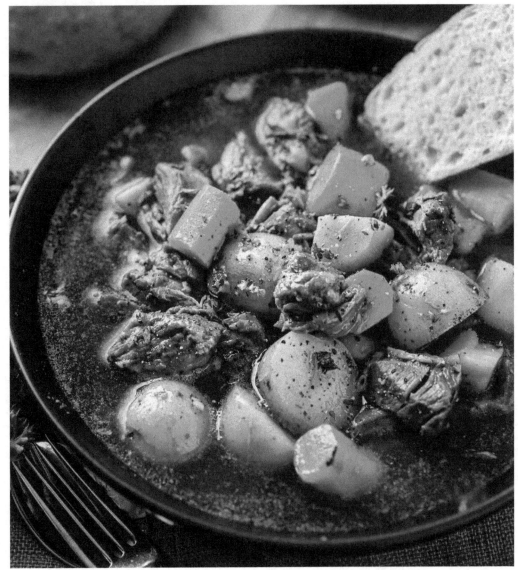

Preparation time: 10 minutes
Cooking time: 6 hours and 10 minutes
Servings: 2

Ingredients:
- 1 tablespoon olive oil
- 1 red onion, chopped
- 1 carrot, peeled and sliced
- 1 pound beef meat, cubed
- ½ cup beef stock
- ½ cup canned tomatoes, chopped

- 2 tablespoons tomato sauce
- 2 tablespoons balsamic vinegar
- 2 garlic cloves, minced
- ½ cup black olives, pitted and sliced
- 1 tablespoon rosemary, chopped
- Salt and black pepper to the taste

Directions:
1. Heat up a pan with the oil over medium-high heat, add the meat, brown for 10 minutes and transfer to your slow cooker.
2. Add the rest of the ingredients, toss, put the lid on and cook on High for 6 hours.
3. Divide between plates and serve right away!

Nutrition: calories 370, fat 14, fiber 6, carbs 26, protein 38

Honey Lamb Roast

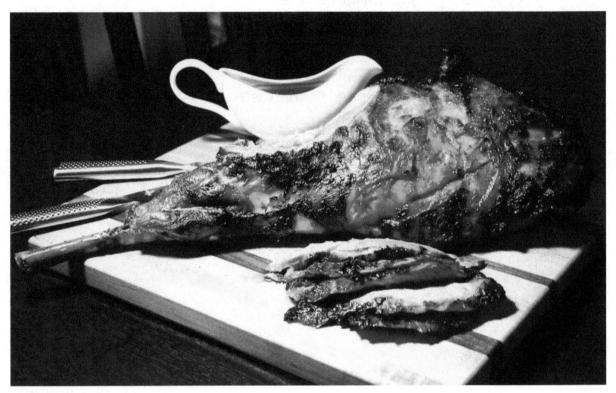

Preparation time: 10 minutes
Cooking time: 7 hours
Servings: 2

Ingredients:

- 1 pound lamb roast, sliced
- 3 tablespoons honey
- ½ tablespoon basil, dried
- ½ tablespoons oregano, dried
- 1 tablespoon garlic, minced
- 1 tablespoon olive oil
- Salt and black pepper to the taste
- ½ cup beef stock

Directions:

1. In your slow cooker, mix the lamb roast with the honey, basil and the other ingredients, toss well, put the lid on and cook on Low for 7 hours.

2. Divide everything between plates and serve.

Nutrition: calories 374, fat 6, fiber 8, carbs 29, protein 6

Beef Strips

Preparation time: 10 minutes
Cooking time: 6 hours
Servings: 4

Ingredients:
- ½ pound baby mushrooms, sliced
- 1 yellow onion, chopped
- 1 pound beef sirloin steak, cubed
- Salt and black pepper to the taste
- 1/3 cup red wine
- 2 teaspoons olive oil
- 2 cups beef stock
- 1 tablespoon Worcestershire sauce

Directions:
1. In your Slow cooker, mix beef strips with onion, mushrooms, salt, pepper, wine, olive oil, beef stock and Worcestershire sauce, toss, cover and cook on Low for 6 hours.
2. Divide between plates and serve for lunch.

Nutrition: calories 212, fat 7, fiber 1, carbs 8, protein 26

Chickpeas Stew

Preparation time: 10 minutes
Cooking time: 6 hours
Servings: 2

Ingredients:
- ½ tablespoon olive oil
- 1 red onion, chopped
- 2 garlic cloves, minced
- 1 red chili pepper, chopped
- ¼ cup carrots, chopped
- 6 ounces canned tomatoes, chopped
- 6 ounces canned chickpeas, drained
- ½ cup chicken stock
- 1 bay leaf
- ½ teaspoon coriander, ground
- A pinch of red pepper flakes
- ½ tablespoon parsley, chopped
- Salt and black pepper to the taste

Directions:
1. In your slow cooker, mix the chickpeas with the onion, garlic and the other ingredients, toss, put the lid on and cook on Low for 6 hours.
2. Divide into bowls and serve.

Nutrition: calories 462, fat 7, fiber 9, carbs 30, protein 17

Fall Slow Cooker Roast

Preparation time: 10 minutes
Cooking time: 6 hours
Servings: 6

Ingredients:

- 2 sweet potatoes, cubed
- 2 carrots, chopped
- 2 pounds beef chuck roast, cubed
- ¼ cup celery, chopped
- 1 tablespoon canola oil
- 2 garlic cloves, minced
- 1 yellow onion, chopped
- 1 tablespoon flour
- 1 tablespoon brown sugar
- 1 tablespoon sugar
- 1 teaspoon cumin, ground
- Salt and black pepper to the taste
- ¾ teaspoon coriander, ground
- ½ teaspoon oregano, dried
- 1 teaspoon chili powder
- 1/8 teaspoon cinnamon powder
- ¾ teaspoon orange peel grated
- 15 ounces tomato sauce

Directions:

1. In your Slow cooker, mix potatoes with carrots, beef cubes, celery, oil, garlic, onion, flour, brown sugar, sugar, cumin, salt pepper, coriander, oregano, chili powder, cinnamon, orange peel and tomato sauce, stir, cover and cook on Low for 6 hours.
2. Divide into bowls and serve for lunch.

Nutrition: calories 278, fat 12, fiber 2, carbs 16, protein 25

Lentils Soup

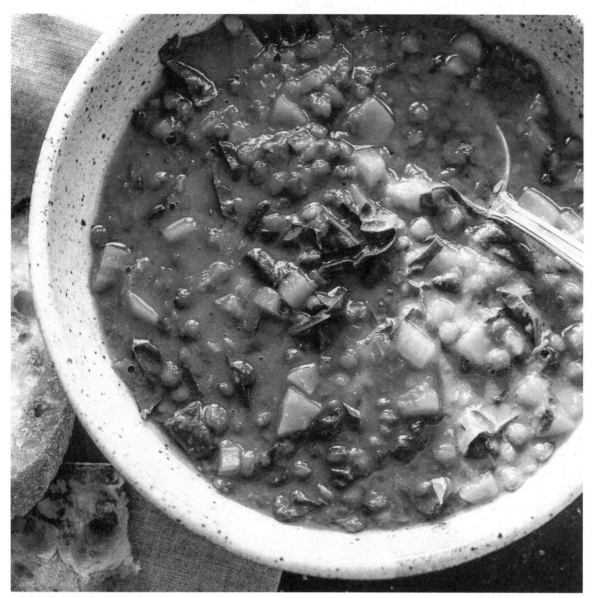

Preparation time: 10 minutes
Cooking time: 4 hours
Servings: 2

Ingredients:

- 2 garlic cloves, minced
- 1 carrot, chopped
- 1 red onion, chopped
- 3 cups veggie stock

- 1 cup brown lentils
- ½ teaspoon cumin, ground
- 1 bay leaf
- 1 tablespoon lime juice
- 1 tablespoon cilantro, chopped
- Salt and black pepper to the taste

Directions:
1. In your slow cooker, mix the lentils with the garlic, carrot and the other ingredients, toss, put the lid on and cook on High for 4 hours.
2. Ladle the soup into bowls and serve.

Nutrition: calories 361, fat 7, fiber 7, carbs 16, protein 5

Creamy Chicken

Preparation time: 10 minutes
Cooking time: 8 hours and 30 minutes
Servings: 6

Ingredients:
- 10 ounces canned cream of chicken soup
- Salt and black pepper to the taste
- A pinch of cayenne pepper
- 3 tablespoons flour
- 1 pound chicken breasts, skinless, boneless and cubed
- 1 celery rib, chopped
- ½ cup green bell pepper, chopped
- ¼ cup yellow onion, chopped
- 10 ounces peas
- 2 tablespoons pimientos, chopped

Directions:
1. In your Slow cooker, mix cream of chicken with salt, pepper, cayenne and flour and whisk well.
2. Add chicken, celery, bell pepper and onion, toss, cover and cook on Low for 8 hours.
3. Add peas and pimientos, stir, cover and cook on Low for 30 minutes more.
4. Divide into bowls and serve for lunch.

Nutrition: calories 200, fat 3, fiber 4, carbs 16, protein 17

Chicken Soup

Preparation time: 10 minutes
Cooking time: 7 hours
Servings: 2

Ingredients:
- ½ pound chicken breast, skinless, boneless and cubed
- 3 cups chicken stock
- 1 red onion, chopped
- 1 garlic clove, minced
- ½ celery stalk, chopped
- ¼ teaspoon chili powder
- ¼ teaspoon sweet paprika
- A pinch of salt and black pepper
- A pinch of cayenne pepper
- 1 tablespoon lemon juice
- ½ tablespoon chives, chopped

Directions:
1. In your slow cooker, mix the chicken with the stock, onion and the other ingredients, toss, put the lid on and cook on Low for 7 hours.
2. Divide into bowls and serve right away.

Nutrition: calories 351, fat 6, fiber 7, carbs 17, protein 16

Chicken Stew

Preparation time: 10 minutes
Cooking time: 8 hours
Servings: 6

Ingredients:
- 32 ounces chicken stock
- 3 spicy chicken sausage links, cooked and sliced
- 28 ounces canned tomatoes, chopped
- 1 yellow onion, chopped
- 1 cup lentils
- 1 carrot, chopped
- 2 garlic cloves, minced
- 1 celery rib, chopped
- ½ teaspoon thyme, dried
- Salt and black pepper to the taste

Directions:
1. In your Slow cooker, mix stock with sausage, tomatoes, onion, lentils, carrot, garlic, celery, thyme, salt and pepper, stir, cover and cook on Low for 8 hours.
2. Divide into bowls and serve for lunch.

Nutrition: calories 231, fat 4, fiber 12, carbs 31, protein 15

Lime and Thyme Chicken

Preparation time: 10 minutes
Cooking time: 6 hours
Servings: 2

Ingredients:
- 1 pound chicken thighs, boneless and skinless
- Juice of 1 lime
- 1 tablespoon lime zest, grated
- 2 teaspoons olive oil
- ½ cup tomato sauce
- 2 garlic cloves, minced
- 1 tablespoon thyme, chopped
- Salt and black pepper to the taste

Directions:
1. In your slow cooker, mix the chicken with the lime juice, zest and the other ingredients, toss, put the lid on and cook on High for 6 hours.
2. Divide between plates and serve right away.

Nutrition: calories 324, fat 7, fiber 8, carbs 20, protein 17

Lemon Chicken

Preparation time: 10 minutes
Cooking time: 5 hours
Servings: 6

Ingredients:
- 6 chicken breast halves, skinless and bone in
- Salt and black pepper to the taste
- 1 teaspoon oregano, dried
- ¼ cup water
- 2 tablespoons butter
- 3 tablespoons lemon juice
- 2 garlic cloves, minced
- 1 teaspoon chicken bouillon granules
- 2 teaspoons parsley, chopped

Directions:
1. In your Slow cooker, mix chicken with salt, pepper, water, butter, lemon juice, garlic and chicken granules, stir, cover and cook on Low for 5 hours.
2. Add parsley, stir, divide between plates and serve for lunch.

Nutrition: calories 336, fat 10, fiber 1, carbs 1, protein 46

Shrimp Gumbo

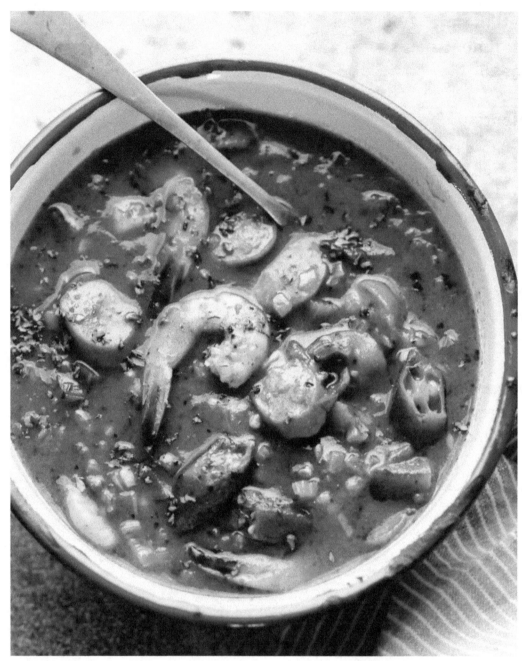

Preparation time: 10 minutes
Cooking time: 2 hours
Servings: 2

Ingredients:
- 1 pound shrimp, peeled and deveined

- ½ pound pork sausage, sliced
- 1 red onion, chopped
- ½ green bell pepper, chopped
- 1 red chili pepper, minced
- ½ teaspoon cumin, ground
- ½ teaspoon coriander, ground
- Salt and black pepper to the taste
- 1 cup tomato sauce
- ½ cup chicken stock
- ½ tablespoon Cajun seasoning
- ½ teaspoon oregano, dried

Directions:

1. In your slow cooker, mix the shrimp with the sausage, onion and the other ingredients, toss, put the lid on and cook on High for 2 hours.
2. Divide into bowls and serve.

Nutrition: calories 721, fat 36.7, fiber 3.7, carbs 18.2, protein 76.6

Chicken Noodle Soup

Preparation time: 10 minutes
Cooking time: 6 hours and 15 minutes
Servings: 4

Ingredients:
- 1 and ½ pound chicken breast, boneless, skinless and cubed
- 1 yellow onion, chopped
- 3 carrots, chopped
- 2 celery stalks, chopped
- 3 garlic cloves minced
- 2 bay leaves
- 1 cup water
- 6 cups chicken stock
- 1 teaspoon Italian seasoning
- 2 cup cheese tortellini
- 1 tablespoon parsley, chopped

Directions:
1. In your Slow cooker, mix chicken with onion, carrots, celery, garlic, bay leaves, water, stock and seasoning, stir, cover and cook on Low for 6 hours.
2. Add tortellini, stir, cover, cook on Low for 15 minutes more, ladle into bowls and serve for lunch.

Nutrition: calories 231, fat 3, fiber 4, carbs 17, protein 22

Squash and Chicken Soup

Preparation time: 10 minutes
Cooking time: 6 hours
Servings: 2

Ingredients:
- ½ pound chicken thighs, skinless, boneless and cubed
- ½ small yellow onion, chopped
- ½ red bell pepper, chopped
- ½ green bell pepper, chopped
- 3 cups chicken stock
- ½ cup butternut squash, peeled and cubed
- 2 ounces canned green chilies, chopped
- ½ teaspoon oregano, dried
- A pinch of salt and black pepper
- ½ tablespoon lime juice
- 1 tablespoon cilantro, chopped

Directions:
1. In your slow cooker, mix the chicken with the onion, bell pepper and the other ingredients, toss, put the lid on and cook on High for 6 hours.
2. Ladle the soup into bowls and serve.

Nutrition: calories 365, fat 11.2, fiber 10.2, carbs 31.4, protein 38

Lentils Soup

Preparation time: 10 minutes
Cooking time: 6 hours
Servings: 6

Ingredients:

- 1 yellow onion, chopped
- 6 carrots, sliced
- 1 yellow bell pepper, chopped
- 4 garlic cloves, minced
- A pinch of cayenne pepper
- 3 cups red lentils
- 4 cups chicken stock
- Salt and black pepper to the taste
- 2 cups water
- 1 teaspoon lemon zest, grated
- 1 teaspoon lemon juice
- 1 tablespoon rosemary, chopped

Directions:

1. In your Slow cooker, mix onion with carrots, bell pepper, garlic, cayenne, lentils, stock, salt, pepper and water, stir, cover and cook on Low for 6 hours.
2. Add lemon zest, lemon juice and rosemary, stir, ladle into bowls and serve for lunch.

Nutrition: calories 281, fat 4, fiber 3, carbs 38, protein 17

Pork Soup

Preparation time: 10 minutes
Cooking time: 6 hours
Servings: 2

Ingredients:
- ½ cup canned black beans, drained and rinsed
- 1 pound pork stew meat, cubed
- 3 cups beef stock
- 1 small red bell pepper, chopped
- 1 yellow onion, chopped
- 1 teaspoon Italian seasoning
- ½ tablespoon olive oil
- Salt and black pepper to the taste
- ½ cup canned tomatoes, crushed
- 1 tablespoon basil, chopped

Directions:
1. In your slow cooker, mix the pork with the beans, stock and the other ingredients, toss, put the lid on and cook on Low for 6 hours.
2. Divide into bowls and serve.

Nutrition: calories 758, fat 27.9, fiber 9.9, carbs 42.1, protein 82.6

Taco Soup

Preparation time: 10 minutes
Cooking time: 6 hours
Servings: 4

Ingredients:
- 1 tablespoon olive oil
- 4 red bell peppers, chopped
- 1 yellow onion, chopped
- 2 pounds beef, ground
- 2 tablespoons chili powder
- 2 tablespoons cumin, ground
- Salt and black pepper to the taste
- 1 teaspoon cinnamon powder
- 1 teaspoon sweet paprika
- ½ teaspoon onion powder
- ½ teaspoon garlic powder
- A pinch of cayenne pepper
- 24 ounces beef stock
- 28 ounces canned tomatoes, chopped
- 8 ounces canned green chilies, chopped
- 6 ounces coconut milk

Directions:
1. In your Slow cooker, mix oil with bell peppers, onion, beef, chili powder, cumin, salt, pepper, cinnamon, paprika, onion powder, garlic powder, cayenne, stock, tomatoes chilies and coconut milk, stir well, cover and cook on Low for 6 hours.
2. Ladle into bowls and serve for lunch.

Nutrition: calories 403, fat 12, fiber 4, carbs 14, protein 45

Mushroom Stew

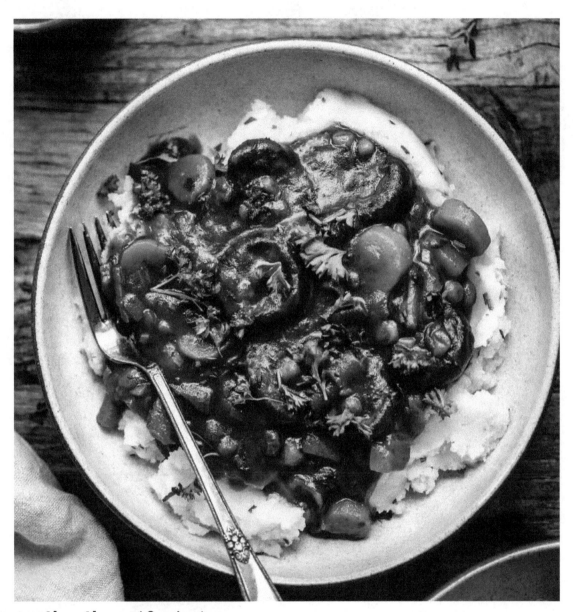

Preparation time: 10 minutes
Cooking time: 6 hours
Servings: 2

Ingredients:

- 1 pound white mushrooms, sliced
- 2 carrots, peeled and cubed
- 1 red onion, chopped
- 1 tablespoon olive oil

- 1 tablespoon balsamic vinegar
- ½ cup tomato sauce
- Salt and black pepper to the taste
- 1 cup veggie stock
- 1 tablespoon basil, chopped

Directions:
1. In your slow cooker, mix the mushrooms with the onion and the other ingredients, toss, put the lid on and cook on Low for 6 hours.
2. Divide the stew into bowls and serve.

Nutrition: calories 400, fat 15, fiber 4, carbs 25, protein 14

Thai Chicken Soup

Preparation time: 10 minutes
Cooking time: 7 hours
Servings: 4

Ingredients:
- 1 pound chicken breasts, skinless and boneless
- 1 cup wild rice
- 1 tablespoon olive oil
- 1 sweet potato, peeled and cubed
- 1 cup butternut squash, peeled and cubed
- 1 zucchini, chopped
- 1 green apple, cored and chopped
- 1 yellow onion, chopped
- 1 tablespoon ginger, grated
- ¼ cup red curry paste
- 4 garlic cloves, minced
- 2 tablespoons brown sugar
- 2 tablespoons fish sauce
- 2 tablespoons soy sauce
- 1 tablespoon basil, dried
- 1 teaspoon cumin, ground
- Salt and black pepper to the taste
- 28 ounces coconut milk
- 5 cups chicken stock

Directions:
1. In your Slow cooker, mix chicken with rice, oil, sweet potato, squash, zucchini, apple, onion, ginger, curry paste, garlic, sugar, fish, soy sauce, basil, cumin, salt, pepper, coconut milk and stock, stir, cover and cook on Low for 7 hours.
2. Transfer meat to a cutting board, shred using 2 forks, return to slow cooker, stir, ladle soup into bowls and serve for lunch.

Nutrition: calories 300, fat 4, fiber 6, carbs 28, protein 17

Beans Chili

Preparation time: 10 minutes
Cooking time: 3 hours
Servings: 2

Ingredients:
- ½ red bell pepper, chopped
- ½ green bell pepper, chopped
- 1 garlic clove, minced
- ½ cup yellow onion, chopped
- ½ cup roasted tomatoes, crushed
- 1 cup canned red kidney beans, drained
- 1 cup canned white beans, drained
- 1 cup canned black beans, drained
- ½ cup corn
- Salt and black pepper to the taste
- 1 tablespoon chili powder
- 1 cup veggie stock

Directions:
1. In your slow cooker, mix the peppers with the beans and the other ingredients, toss, put the lid on and cook on High for 3 hours.
2. Divide into bowls and serve right away.

Nutrition: calories 400, fat 14, fiber 5, carbs 29, protein 22

Spinach and Mushroom Soup

Preparation time: 10 minutes
Cooking time: 3 hours
Servings: 6

Ingredients:
- 2/3 cup yellow onion, chopped
- 16 ounces baby spinach
- 3 tablespoons butter
- Salt and black pepper to the taste
- 5 cups veggie stock
- 3 garlic cloves, minced
- ½ teaspoon Italian seasoning
- 1 and ½ cups half and half
- ¼ teaspoon thyme, dried
- 16 ounces cheese tortellini
- 2 teaspoons garlic powder
- 3 cups mushrooms, sliced
- ½ cup parmesan, grated

Directions:
1. Heat up a pan with the butter over medium-high heat, add onion, garlic, mushrooms and spinach, stir and cook for a few minutes.
2. Transfer to your Slow cooker, add salt, pepper, stock, Italian seasoning, half and half, thyme, garlic powder and parmesan, cover and cook on High for 2 hours and 30 minutes.
3. Add tortellini, stir, cover, cook on High for 30 minutes more, ladle into bowls and serve for lunch.

Nutrition: calories 231, fat 5, fiber 6, carbs 14, protein 5

Parsley Chicken Stew

Preparation time: 10 minutes
Cooking time: 4 hours
Servings: 2

Ingredients:
- 1 tablespoon olive oil
- Salt and black pepper to the taste
- 2 spring onions, chopped
- 1 carrot, peeled and sliced
- ¼ cup chicken stock
- 1 pound chicken breast, skinless, boneless sand cubed
- ½ cup tomato sauce
- 1 tablespoon parsley, chopped

Directions:
1. In your slow cooker, mix the chicken with the spring onions and the other ingredients, toss, put the lid on and cook on High for 4 hours.
2. Divide into bowls and serve.

Nutrition: calories 453, fat 15, fiber 5, carbs 20, protein 20

Creamy Chicken Soup

Preparation time: 10 minutes
Cooking time: 6 hours
Servings: 6

Ingredients:
- 2 chicken breasts, skinless and boneless
- 1 cup yellow corn
- 1 cup peas
- 1 celery stalk, chopped
- 1 cup carrots, chopped
- 2 gold potatoes, cubed
- 4 ounces cream cheese, soft
- 1 yellow onion, chopped
- 4 cups chicken stock
- 2 teaspoons garlic powder
- 3 cups heavy cream
- Salt and black pepper to the taste

Directions:
1. In your Slow cooker, mix chicken with corn, peas, carrots, potatoes, celery, cream cheese, onion, garlic powder, stock, heavy cream, salt and pepper, stir, cover and cook on Low for 6 hours.
2. Transfer chicken to a cutting board, shred meat using 2 forks, return to the slow cooker, stir, ladle soup into bowls and serve for lunch.

Nutrition: calories 300, fat 6, fiber 5, carbs 20, protein 22

Mustard Short Ribs

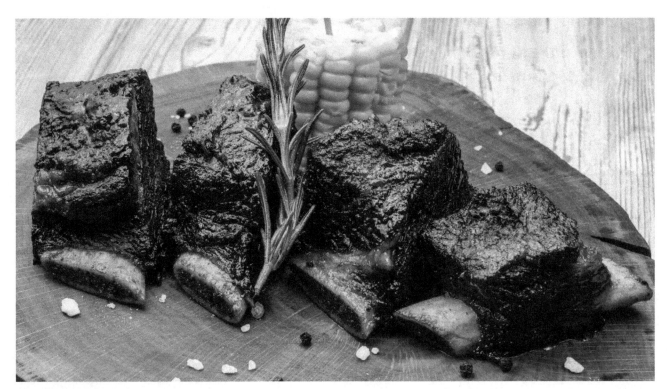

Preparation time: 10 minutes
Cooking time: 8 hours
Servings: 2

Ingredients:
- 2 beef short ribs, bone in and cut into individual ribs
- Salt and black pepper to the taste
- ½ cup BBQ sauce
- 1 tablespoon mustard
- 1 tablespoon green onions, chopped

Directions:
1. In your slow cooker, mix the ribs with the sauce and the other ingredients, toss, put the lid on and cook on Low for 8 hours.
2. Divide the mix between plates and serve.

Nutrition: calories 284, fat 7, 4, carbs 18, protein 20

Black Bean Soup

Preparation time: 10 minutes
Cooking time: 6 hours
Servings: 6

Ingredients:
- 1 pound black beans
- 2 celery stalks, chopped
- 2 garlic cloves, minced
- 1 yellow onion, chopped
- 2 carrots, chopped
- 1 tablespoon chili powder
- 1 cup salsa
- 1 teaspoon oregano, dried
- ½ tablespoon cumin, ground
- 2 cups water
- 4 cups veggie stock

Directions:
1. In your Slow cooker, mix beans with celery, garlic, onion, carrots, chili powder, salsa, oregano, cumin, water and stock, stir, cover and cook on Low for 6 hours.
2. Blend soup using an immersion blender, ladle into bowls and serve for lunch.

Nutrition: calories 300, fat 4, fiber 7, carbs 20, protein 16

Creamy Brisket

Preparation time: 10 minutes
Cooking time: 8 hours
Servings: 2

Ingredients:
- 1 tablespoon olive oil
- 1 shallot, chopped
- 2 garlic cloves, mined
- 1 pound beef brisket
- Salt and black pepper to the taste
- ¼ cup beef stock
- 3 tablespoons heavy cream
- 1 tablespoon parsley, chopped

Directions:
1. In your slow cooker, mix the brisket with the oil and the other ingredients, toss, put the lid on and cook on Low for 8 hours.
2. Transfer the beef to a cutting board, slice, divide between plates and serve with the sauce drizzled all over.

Nutrition: calories 400, fat 10, fiber 4, carbs 15, protein 20

Winter Veggie Stew

Preparation time: 10 minutes
Cooking time: 4 hours
Servings: 8

Ingredients:
- 1 yellow onion, chopped
- 1 teaspoon olive oil
- 2 red potatoes, chopped
- Salt and black pepper to the taste
- 1 tablespoon sugar
- 1 tablespoon curry powder
- 1 tablespoon ginger, grated
- 3 garlic cloves, minced
- 30 ounces canned chickpeas, drained
- 1 green bell pepper, chopped
- 2 cups chicken stock
- 1 red bell pepper, chopped
- 1 cauliflower head, florets separated
- 28 ounces canned tomatoes, chopped
- 1 cup coconut milk
- 10 ounces baby spinach

Directions:
1. In your slow cooker, mix oil with onion, potatoes, salt, pepper, sugar, curry powder, ginger, garlic, chickpeas, red and green bell pepper, stock, cauliflower, tomatoes, spinach and milk, stir, cover and cook on High for 4 minutes.
2. Stir your stew again, divide into bowls and serve for lunch.

Nutrition: calories 319, fat 10, fiber 13, carbs 45, protein 14

Mushroom Soup

Preparation time: 10 minutes
Cooking time: 4 hours
Servings: 2

Ingredients:
- 1 small yellow onion, chopped
- 1 carrot, chopped
- 1 small red bell pepper, chopped
- 1 green bell pepper, chopped
- 1 pound mushrooms, sliced
- 1 garlic clove, minced
- ½ teaspoon Italian seasoning
- Salt and black pepper to the taste
- 3 cups chicken stock
- ½ cup half and half
- 1 tablespoon chives, chopped

Directions:
1. In your slow cooker, mix the mushrooms with the onion, carrot and the other ingredients, toss, put the lid on and cook on High for 4 hours.
2. Divide into bowls and serve.

Nutrition: calories 453, fat 14, fiber 6, carbs 28, protein 33

Chickpeas Stew

Preparation time: 10 minutes
Cooking time: 4 hours and 10 minutes
Servings: 6

Ingredients:
- 1 yellow onion, chopped
- 1 tablespoon ginger, grated
- 1 tablespoon olive oil
- 6 ounces canned chickpeas, drained
- 4 garlic cloves, minced
- Salt and black pepper to the taste
- 2 red Thai chilies, chopped
- ½ teaspoon turmeric powder
- 2 tablespoons garam masala
- 4 ounces tomato paste
- 2 cups chicken stock
- 2 tablespoons cilantro, chopped

Directions:
1. Heat up a pan with the oil over medium-high heat, add ginger and onions, stir and cook for 4-5 minutes.
2. Add garlic, salt, pepper, Thai chilies, garam masala and turmeric, stir, cook for 2 minutes more and transfer everything to your slow cooker.
3. Add stock, chickpeas and tomato paste, stir, cover and cook on Low for 4 hours.
4. Add cilantro, stir, divide into bowls and serve for lunch.

Nutrition: calories 225, fat 7, fiber 4, carbs 14, protein 7

Creamy Potato Soup

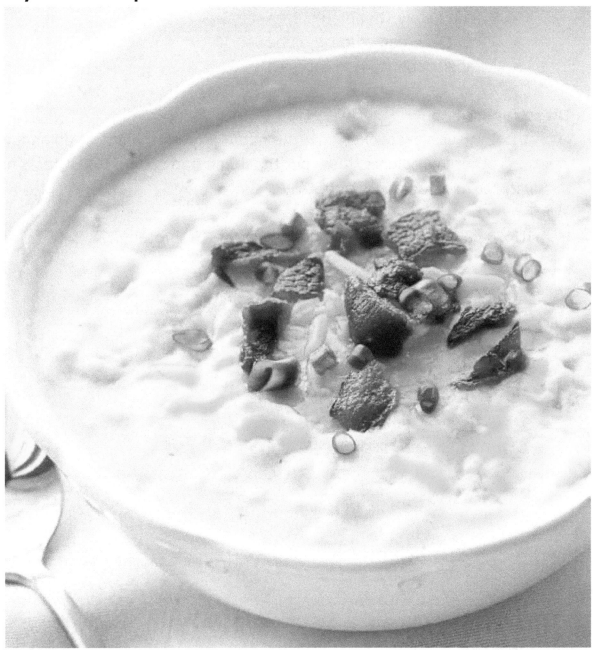

Preparation time: 10 minutes
Cooking time: 5 hours
Servings: 2

Ingredients:

- 1 small yellow onion, chopped
- 3 cups chicken stock
- ½ pound red potatoes, peeled and cubed

51

- 1 teaspoon turmeric powder
- ½ cup heavy whipping cream
- 2 ounces cream cheese, cubed
- 1 tablespoon chives, chopped

Directions:

1. In your slow cooker, mix the potatoes with the stock, onion and the other ingredients, toss, put the lid on and cook on High for 5 hours.
2. Divide into bowls and serve.

Nutrition: calories 372, fat 15, fiber 4, carbs 20, protein 22

Lentils Curry

Preparation time: 10 minutes
Cooking time: 8 hours
Servings: 16

Ingredients:
- 4 garlic cloves, minced
- 4 cups brown lentils
- 2 yellow onions, chopped
- 1 tablespoon ginger, grated
- 4 tablespoons olive oil
- 1 tablespoon garam masala
- 4 tablespoons red curry paste
- 2 teaspoons sugar
- 1 and ½ teaspoons turmeric powder
- A pinch of salt and black pepper
- 45 ounces canned tomato puree
- ½ cup coconut milk
- 1 tablespoon cilantro, chopped

Directions:
1. In your slow cooker, mix lentils with onions, garlic, ginger, oil, curry paste, garam masala, turmeric, salt, pepper, sugar and tomato puree, stir, cover and cook on Low for 7 hours and 20 minutes.
2. Add coconut milk and cilantro, stir, cover, cook on Low for 40 minutes, divide into bowls and serve for lunch.

Nutrition: calories 268, fat 5, fiber 4, carbs 18, protein 6

Chicken with Corn and Wild Rice

Preparation time: 10 minutes
Cooking time: 6 hours
Servings: 2

Ingredients:
- 1 pound chicken breast, skinless, boneless and cubed
- 1 cup wild rice
- 1 cup chicken stock
- 1 tablespoon tomato paste
- Salt and black pepper to the taste
- ¼ teaspoon cumin, ground
- 3 ounces canned roasted tomatoes, chopped
- ¼ cup corn
- 2 tablespoons cilantro, chopped

Directions:
1. In your slow cooker, mix the chicken with the rice, stock and the other ingredients, toss, put the lid on and cook on Low for 6 hours.
2. Divide everything between plates and serve.

Nutrition: calories 372, fat 12, fiber 5, carbs 20, protein 25

Quinoa Chili

Preparation time: 10 minutes
Cooking time: 3 hours
Servings: 4

Ingredients:
- 15 ounces canned black beans, drained
- 2 and ¼ cups veggie stock
- ½ cup quinoa
- 14 ounces canned tomatoes, chopped
- ¼ cup red bell pepper, chopped
- 1 carrot, sliced
- ¼ cup green bell pepper, chopped
- 2 garlic cloves, minced
- ½ chili pepper, chopped
- ½ cup corn
- 2 teaspoons chili powder
- 1 small yellow onion, chopped
- Salt and black pepper to the taste
- 1 teaspoon oregano, dried
- 1 teaspoon cumin, ground

Directions:
1. In your slow cooker, mix black beans with stock, quinoa, tomatoes, red and green bell pepper, carrot, garlic, chili, chili powder, onion, salt, pepper, oregano, cumin and corn, stir, cover and cook on High for 3 hours.
2. Divide chili into bowls and serve for lunch.

Nutrition: calories 291, fat 7, fiber 4, carbs 28, protein 8

Mixed Pork and Beans

Preparation time: 10 minutes
Cooking time: 8 hours
Servings: 2

Ingredients:
- 1 cup canned black beans, drained
- 1 cup green beans, trimmed and halved
- ½ pound pork shoulder, cubed
- Salt and black pepper to the taste
- 3 garlic cloves, minced
- ½ yellow onion, chopped
- ½ cup beef stock
- ¼ tablespoon balsamic vinegar
- 1 tablespoon olive oil

Directions:
1. In your slow cooker, mix the beans with the pork and the other ingredients, toss, put the lid on and cook on Low for 8 hours.
2. Divide everything between plates and serve.

Nutrition: calories 453, fat 10, fiber 12, carbs 20, protein 36

French Veggie Stew

Preparation time: 10 minutes
Cooking time: 9 hours
Servings: 6

Ingredients:
- 2 yellow onions, chopped
- 1 eggplant, sliced
- 4 zucchinis, sliced
- 2 garlic cloves, minced
- 2 green bell peppers, cut into medium strips
- 6 ounces canned tomato paste
- 2 tomatoes, cut into medium wedges
- 1 teaspoon oregano, dried
- 1 teaspoon sugar
- 1 teaspoon basil, dried
- Salt and black pepper to the taste
- 2 tablespoons parsley, chopped
- ¼ cup olive oil
- A pinch of red pepper flakes, crushed

Directions:
1. In your Slow cooker, mix oil with onions, eggplant, zucchinis, garlic, bell peppers, tomato paste, basil, sugar, oregano, salt and pepper, cover and cook on Low for 9 hours.
2. Add pepper flakes and parsley, stir gently, divide into bowls and serve for lunch.

Nutrition: calories 269, fat 7, fiber 6, carbs 17, protein 4

Pork Chops and Butter Sauce

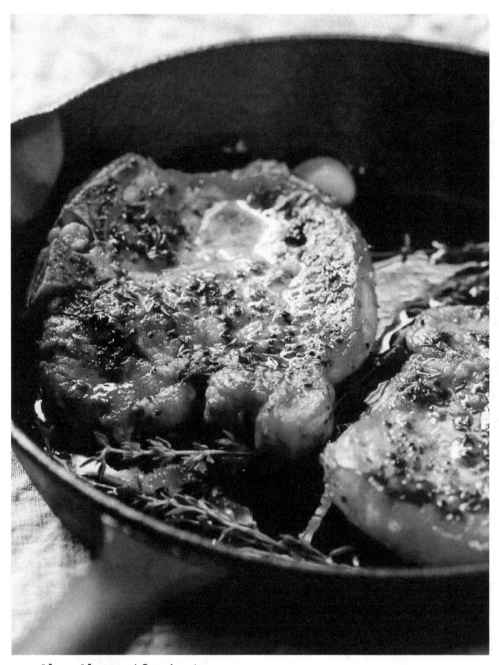

Preparation time: 10 minutes
Cooking time: 7 hours
Servings: 2

Ingredients:
- ½ pound pork loin chops
- 2 tablespoons butter

- 2 scallions, chopped
- 1 cup beef stock
- 1 garlic clove, minced
- ¼ teaspoon thyme, dried
- Salt and black pepper to the taste
- ¼ cup heavy cream
- ¼ tablespoon cornstarch
- ½ teaspoon basil, dried

Directions:
1. In your slow cooker, mix the pork chops with the butter, scallions and the other ingredients, toss, put the lid on and cook on Low for 7 hours.
2. Divide everything between plates and serve.

Nutrition: calories 453, fat 16, fiber 8, carbs 7, protein 27

Beans and Rice

Preparation time: 10 minutes
Cooking time: 3 hours
Servings: 6

Ingredients:
- 1 pound pinto beans, dried
- 1/3 cup hot sauce
- Salt and black pepper to the taste
- 1 tablespoon garlic, minced
- 1 teaspoon garlic powder
- ½ teaspoon cumin, ground
- 1 tablespoon chili powder
- 3 bay leaves
- ½ teaspoon oregano, dried
- 1 cup white rice, cooked

Directions:
1. In your slow cooker, mix pinto beans with hot sauce, salt, pepper, garlic, garlic powder, cumin, chili powder, bay leaves and oregano, stir, cover and cook on High for 3 hours.
2. Divide rice between plates, add pinto beans on top and serve for lunch

Nutrition: calories 381, fat 7, fiber 12, carbs 35, protein 10

Chicken and Peach Mix

Preparation time: 10 minutes
Cooking time: 6 hours
Servings: 2

Ingredients:
- 1 pound chicken breast, skinless and boneless
- 1 cup peaches, cubed
- ½ tablespoon avocado oil
- ½ cup chicken stock
- 1 tablespoon balsamic vinegar
- ½ teaspoon garlic, minced
- ¼ cup cherry tomatoes, halved
- 1 tablespoon basil, chopped

Directions:
1. In your slow cooker, mix the chicken with the peaches, oil and the other ingredients, toss, put the lid on and cook on Low for 6 hours.
2. Divide everything between plates and serve.

Nutrition: calories 300, fat 7, fiber 8, carbs 20, protein 39

Black Beans Stew

Preparation time: 10 minutes
Cooking time: 6 hours and 20 minutes
Servings: 6

Ingredients:
- 1 yellow onion, chopped
- 1 tablespoon olive oil
- 1 red bell pepper, chopped
- 1 jalapeno, chopped
- 2 garlic cloves, minced
- 1 teaspoon ginger, grated
- ½ teaspoon cumin
- ½ teaspoon allspice, ground
- ½ teaspoon oregano, dried
- 30 ounces canned black beans, drained
- ½ teaspoon sugar
- 1 cup chicken stock
- Salt and black pepper
- 3 cups brown rice, cooked
- 2 mangoes, peeled and chopped

Directions:
1. Heat up a pan with the oil over medium-high heat, add onion, stir and cook for 3-4 minutes,
2. Add garlic, ginger and jalapeno, stir, cook for 3 minutes more and transfer to your slow cooker.
3. Add red bell pepper, cumin, allspice, oregano, black beans, sugar, stock, salt and pepper, stir, cover and cook on Low for 6 hours.
4. Add rice and mangoes, stir, cover, cook on Low for 10 minutes more, divide between plates and serve.

Nutrition: calories 490, fat 6, fiber 20, carbs 80, protein 17

Chicken Drumsticks and Buffalo Sauce

Preparation time: 10 minutes
Cooking time: 8 hours
Servings: 2

Ingredients:
- 1 pound chicken drumsticks
- 2 tablespoons buffalo wing sauce
- ½ cup chicken stock
- 2 tablespoons honey
- 1 teaspoon lemon juice
- Salt and black pepper to the taste

Directions:
1. In your slow cooker, mix the chicken with the sauce and the other ingredients, toss, put the lid on and cook on Low for 8 hours.
2. Divide everything between plates and serve.

Nutrition: calories 361, fat 7, fiber 8, carbs 18, protein 22

Sweet Potato Stew

Preparation time: 10 minutes
Cooking time: 8 hours
Servings: 8

Ingredients:
- 1 yellow onion, chopped
- ½ cup red beans, dried
- 2 red bell peppers, chopped
- 2 tablespoons ginger, grated
- 4 garlic cloves, minced
- 2 pounds sweet, peeled and cubed
- 3 cups chicken stock
- 14 ounces canned tomatoes, chopped
- 2 jalapeno peppers, chopped
- Salt and black pepper to the taste
- ½ teaspoon cumin, ground
- ½ teaspoon coriander, ground
- ¼ teaspoon cinnamon powder
- ¼ cup peanuts, roasted and chopped
- Juice of ½ lime

Directions:
1. In your slow cooker, mix onion with red beans, red bell peppers, ginger, garlic, potatoes, stock, tomatoes, jalapenos, salt, pepper, cumin, coriander and cinnamon, stir, cover and cook on Low for 8 hours.
2. Divide into bowls, divide peanuts on top, drizzle lime juice and serve for lunch.

Nutrition: calories 259, fat 8, fiber 7, carbs 42, protein 8

Mustard Pork Chops and Carrots

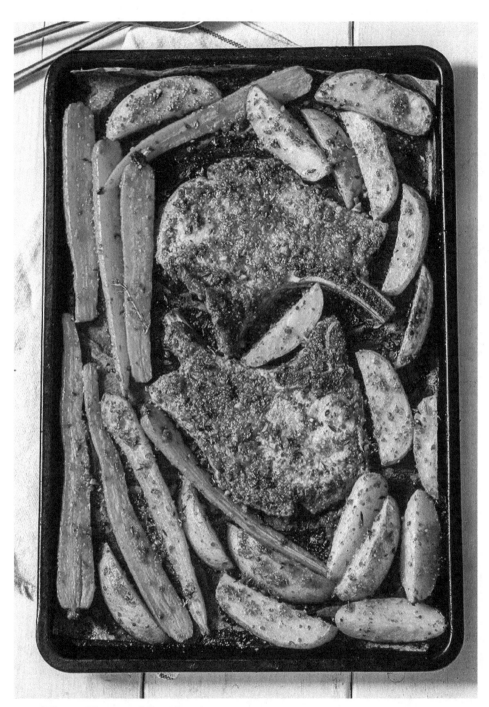

Preparation time: 10 minutes
Cooking time: 4 hours
Servings: 2

Ingredients:

- 1 tablespoon butter
- 1 pound pork chops, bone in
- 2 carrots, sliced
- 1 cup beef stock
- ½ tablespoon honey
- ½ tablespoon lime juice
- 1 tablespoon lime zest, grated

Directions:

1. In your slow cooker, mix the pork chops with the butter and the other ingredients, toss, put the lid on and cook on High for 4 hours.
2. Divide between plate sand serve.

Nutrition: calories 300, fat 8, fiber 10, carbs 16, protein 16

Minestrone Soup

Preparation time: 10 minutes
Cooking time: 4 hours
Servings: 8

Ingredients:
- 2 zucchinis, chopped
- 3 carrots, chopped
- 1 yellow onion, chopped
- 1 cup green beans, halved
- 3 celery stalks, chopped
- 4 garlic cloves, minced
- 10 ounces canned garbanzo beans
- 1 pound lentils, cooked
- 4 cups veggie stock
- 28 ounces canned tomatoes, chopped
- 1 teaspoon curry powder
- ½ teaspoon garam masala
- ½ teaspoon cumin, ground
- Salt and black pepper to the taste

Directions:
1. In your slow cooker, mix zucchinis with carrots, onion, green beans, celery, garlic, garbanzo beans, lentils, stock, tomatoes, salt, pepper, cumin, curry powder and garam masala, stir, cover, cook on High for 4 hours, ladle into bowls and serve for lunch.

Nutrition: calories 273, fat 12, fiber 7, carbs 34, protein 10

Fennel Soup

Preparation time: 10 minutes
Cooking time: 4 hours
Servings: 2

Ingredients:
- 2 fennel bulbs, sliced
- ½ cup tomatoes, crushed
- 1 red onion, sliced
- 1 leek, chopped
- 2 cups veggie stock
- ½ teaspoon cumin, ground
- 1 tablespoon dill, chopped
- ½ tablespoon olive oil
- Salt and black pepper to the taste

Directions:
1. In your slow cooker, mix the fennel with the tomatoes, onion and the other ingredients, toss, put the lid on and cook on High for 4 hours.
2. Ladle into bowls and serve hot.

Nutrition: calories 132, fat 2, fiber 5, carbs 11, protein 3

Chili Cream

Preparation time: 10 minutes
Cooking time: 6 hours
Servings: 6

Ingredients:
- 2 jalapeno chilies, chopped
- 1 cup yellow onion, chopped
- 1 tablespoon olive oil
- 4 poblano chilies, chopped
- 4 Anaheim chilies, chopped
- 3 cups corn
- 6 cups veggie stock
- ½ bunch cilantro, chopped
- Salt and black pepper to the taste

Directions:
1. In your slow cooker, mix jalapenos with onion, oil, poblano chilies, Anaheim chilies, corn and stock, stir, cover and cook on Low for 6 hours.
2. Add cilantro, salt and pepper, stir, transfer to your blender, pulse well, divide into bowls and serve for lunch.

Nutrition: calories 209, fat 5, fiber 5, carbs 33, protein 5

Artichoke Soup

Preparation time: 10 minutes
Cooking time: 5 hours
Servings: 2

Ingredients:
- 2 cups canned artichoke hearts, drained and halved
- 1 small carrot, chopped
- 1 small yellow onion, chopped
- 1 garlic clove, minced
- ¼ teaspoon oregano, dried
- ¼ teaspoon rosemary, dried
- A pinch of red pepper flakes
- A pinch of garlic powder
- A pinch of salt and black pepper
- 3 cups chicken stock
- 1 tablespoon tomato paste
- 1 tablespoon cilantro, chopped

Directions:
1. In your slow cooker, mix the artichokes with the carrot, onion and the other ingredients, toss, put the lid on and cook on Low for 5 hours.
2. Ladle into bowls and serve.

Nutrition: calories 362, fat 3, fiber 5, carbs 16, protein 5

Salmon and Cilantro Sauce

Preparation time: 10 minutes
Cooking time: 2 hours and 30 minutes
Servings: 4

Ingredients:
- 2 garlic cloves, minced
- 4 salmon fillets, boneless
- ¾ cup cilantro, chopped
- 3 tablespoons lime juice
- 1 tablespoon olive oil
- Salt and black pepper to the taste

Directions:
1. Grease your Slow cooker with the oil, add salmon fillets inside skin side down, also add garlic, cilantro, lime juice, salt and pepper, cover and cook on Low for 2 hours and 30 minutes.
2. Divide salmon fillets on plates, drizzle the cilantro sauce all over and serve for lunch.

Nutrition: calories 200, fat 3, fiber 2, carbs 14, protein 8

Beans and Mushroom Stew

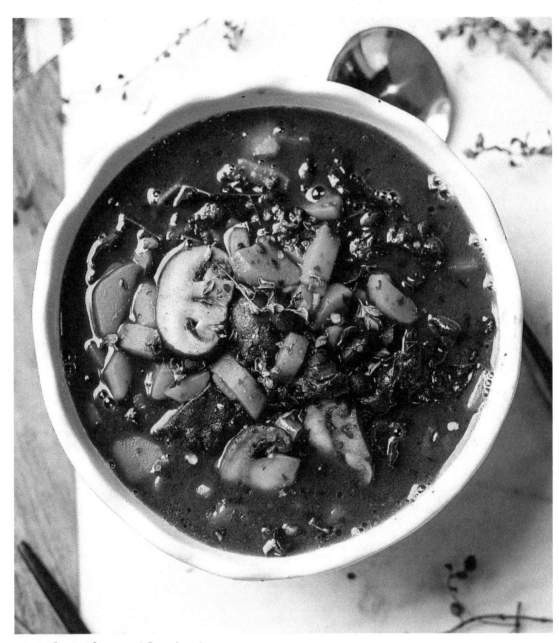

Preparation time: 10 minutes
Cooking time: 8 hours
Servings: 2

Ingredients:

- Cooking spray
- ½ green bell pepper, chopped
- ½ red bell pepper, chopped

- ½ red onion, chopped
- 2 garlic cloves, minced
- 1 cup tomatoes, cubed
- 1 cup veggie stock
- Salt and black pepper to the taste
- 1 cup white mushrooms, sliced
- 1 cup canned kidney beans, drained
- ½ teaspoon turmeric powder
- ½ teaspoon coriander, ground
- 1 tablespoon parsley, chopped
- ½ tablespoon Cajun seasoning

Directions:
1. Grease the slow cooker with the cooking spray and mix the bell peppers with the onion, garlic and the other ingredients into the pot.
2. Put the lid on, cook on Low for 8 hours, divide into bowls and serve.

Nutrition: calories 272, fat 4, fiber 7, carbs 19, protein 7

Chili Salmon

Preparation time: 10 minutes
Cooking time: 2 hours
Servings: 2

Ingredients:
- 2 medium salmon fillets, boneless
- A pinch of nutmeg, ground
- A pinch of cloves, ground
- A pinch of ginger powder
- Salt and black pepper to the taste
- 2 teaspoons sugar
- 1 teaspoon onion powder
- ¼ teaspoon chipotle chili powder
- ½ teaspoon cayenne pepper
- ½ teaspoon cinnamon, ground
- 1/8 teaspoon thyme, dried

Directions:
1. In a bowl, mix salmon fillets with nutmeg, cloves, ginger, salt, coconut sugar, onion powder, chili powder, cayenne black pepper, cinnamon and thyme, toss, transfer fish to 2 tin foil pieces, wrap, add to your Slow cooker, cover and cook on Low for 2 hours.
2. Unwrap fish, divide between plates and serve with a side salad for lunch.

Nutrition: calories 220, fat 4, fiber 2, carbs 7, protein 4

Chicken and Eggplant Stew

Preparation time: 10 minutes
Cooking time: 8 hours
Servings: 2

Ingredients:
- 1 cup tomato paste
- ½ cup chicken stock
- 1 pound chicken breast, skinless, boneless and cubed
- 2 eggplants, cubed
- 1 small red onion, chopped
- 1 red bell pepper, chopped
- ½ teaspoon rosemary, dried
- ½ tablespoon smoked paprika
- 1 teaspoon cumin, ground
- Cooking spray
- Salt and black pepper to the taste
- Juice of ½ lemon
- ½ tablespoon parsley, chopped

Directions:
1. In your slow cooker, mix the chicken with the stock, tomato paste and the other ingredients, toss, put the lid on and cook on Low for 8 hours.
2. Divide into bowls and serve for lunch.

Nutrition: calories 261, fat 4, fiber 6, carbs 14, protein 7

Pulled Chicken

Preparation time: 10 minutes
Cooking time: 6 hours
Servings: 2

Ingredients:
- 2 tomatoes, chopped
- 2 red onions, chopped
- 2 chicken breasts, skinless and boneless
- 2 garlic cloves, minced
- 1 tablespoon maple syrup
- 1 teaspoon chili powder
- 1 teaspoon basil, dried
- 3 tablespoons water
- 1 teaspoon cloves, ground

Directions:
1. In your Slow cooker, mix onion with tomatoes, chicken, garlic, maple syrup, chili powder, basil, water and cloves, toss well, cover and cook on Low for 6 hours.
2. Shred chicken, divide it along with the veggies between plates and serve for lunch.

Nutrition: calories 220, fat 3, fiber 3, carbs 14, protein 6

Turmeric Lentils Stew

Preparation time: 10 minutes
Cooking time: 5 hours
Servings: 2

Ingredients:
- 2 cups veggie stock
- ½ cup canned red lentils, drained
- 1 carrot, sliced
- 1 eggplant, cubed
- ½ cup tomatoes, chopped
- 1 red onion, chopped
- 1 garlic clove, minced
- 1 teaspoon turmeric powder
- ¼ tablespoons ginger, grated
- ½ teaspoons mustard seeds
- ¼ teaspoon sweet paprika
- ½ cup tomato paste
- 1 tablespoon dill, chopped
- Salt and black pepper to the taste

Directions:
1. In your slow cooker, combine the lentils with the stock, tomatoes, eggplant and the other ingredients, toss, put the lid on, cook on High for 5 hours, divide into bowls and serve.

Nutrition: calories 303, fat 4, fiber 8, carbs 12, protein 4

Chicken Chili

Preparation time: 10 minutes
Cooking time: 7 hours
Servings: 4

Ingredients:
- 16 ounces salsa
- 8 chicken thighs
- 1 yellow onion, chopped
- 16 ounces canned tomatoes, chopped
- 1 red bell pepper, chopped
- 2 tablespoons chili powder

Directions:
1. Put the salsa in your slow cooker, add chicken, onion, tomatoes, bell pepper and chili powder, stir, cover, cook on Low for 7 hours, divide into bowls and serve for lunch.

Nutrition: calories 250, fat 3, fiber 3, carbs 14, protein 8

Pork Chili

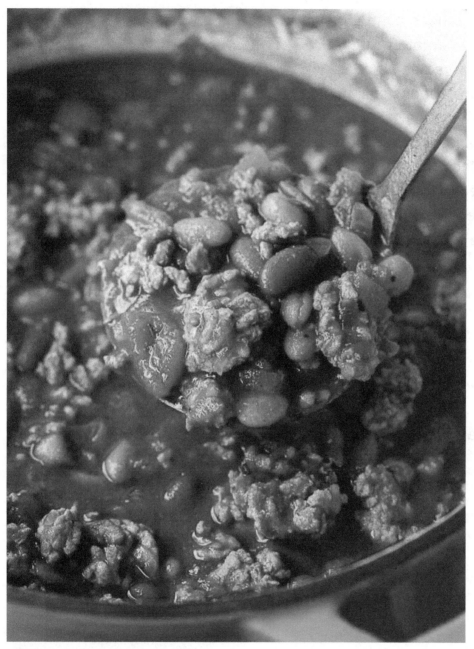

Preparation time: 10 minutes
Cooking time: 10 hours
Servings: 2

Ingredients:

- 1 pound pork stew meat, cubed
- 1 red onion, sliced

- 1 carrot, sliced
- 1 teaspoon sweet paprika
- ½ teaspoon cumin, ground
- 1 cup tomato paste
- 1 cup veggie stock
- 2 tablespoons chili powder
- 2 teaspoons cayenne pepper
- 1 tablespoon red pepper flakes
- A pinch of salt and black pepper
- 1 red bell pepper, chopped
- 1 yellow bell pepper, chopped
- 1 tablespoon chives, chopped

Directions:

1. In your slow cooker, mix the pork meat with the onion, carrot and the other ingredients, toss, put the lid on and cook on Low for 10 hours.
2. Divide the mix into bowls and serve.

Nutrition: calories 261, fat 7, fiber 4, carbs 8, protein 18

Salsa Chicken

Preparation time: 10 minutes
Cooking time: 7 hours
Servings: 4

Ingredients:
- 4 chicken breasts, skinless and boneless
- ½ cup veggie stock
- Salt and black pepper to the taste
- 16 ounces salsa
- 1 and ½ tablespoons parsley, dried
- 1 teaspoon garlic powder
- ½ tablespoon cilantro, chopped
- 1 teaspoon onion powder
- ½ tablespoons oregano, dried
- ½ teaspoon paprika, smoked
- 1 teaspoon chili powder
- ½ teaspoon cumin, ground

Directions:
1. Put the stock in your slow cooker, add chicken breasts, add salsa, parsley, garlic powder, cilantro, onion powder, oregano, paprika, chili powder, cumin, salt and black pepper to the taste, stir, cover and cook on Low for 7 hours.
2. Divide chicken between plates, drizzle the sauces on top and serve for lunch.

Nutrition: calories 270, fat 4, fiber 2, carbs 14, protein 9

Cinnamon Pork Ribs

Preparation time: 10 minutes
Cooking time: 8 hours
Servings: 2

Ingredients:
- 2 pounds baby back pork ribs
- 1 tablespoon cinnamon powder
- 2 tablespoons olive oil
- ½ teaspoon allspice, ground
- A pinch of salt and black pepper
- ½ teaspoon garlic powder
- 1 tablespoon balsamic vinegar
- ½ cup beef stock
- 1 tablespoon tomato paste

Directions:
1. In your slow cooker, mix the pork ribs with the cinnamon, the oil and the other ingredients, toss, put the lid on and cook on Low for 8 hours.
2. Divide ribs between plates and serve for lunch with a side salad.

Nutrition: calories 312, fat 7, fiber 7, carbs 8, protein 18

Thai Chicken

Preparation time: 10 minutes
Cooking time: 4 hours
Servings: 6

Ingredients:
- 1 and ½ pound chicken breast, boneless, skinless and cubed
- 1 tablespoon olive oil
- 3 tablespoons soy sauce
- 2 tablespoons flour
- Salt and black pepper to the taste
- 1 tablespoon ketchup
- 2 tablespoons white vinegar
- 1 teaspoon ginger, grated
- 2 tablespoons sugar
- ½ cup cashews, chopped
- 2 garlic cloves, minced
- 1 green onion, chopped

Directions:
1. Put chicken pieces in a bowl, season with salt, black pepper, add flour and toss well.
2. Heat up a pan with the oil over medium-high heat, add chicken, cook for 5 minutes and transfer to your slow cooker.
3. Add soy sauce, ketchup, vinegar, ginger, sugar and garlic, stir well, cover, cook on Low for 4 hours, add cashews and green onion, stir, divide into bowls and serve for lunch.

Nutrition: calories 200, fat 3, fiber 2, carbs 13, protein 12

Pork and Mushroom Stew

Preparation time: 10 minutes
Cooking time: 7 hours
Servings: 2

Ingredients:
- 2 tablespoons olive oil
- 1 garlic clove, minced
- 1 red onion, sliced
- 2 pounds pork stew meat, cubed
- 1 cup mushrooms, sliced
- 1 cup tomato paste
- A pinch of salt and black pepper
- 1 teaspoon oregano, dried
- 1 teaspoon rosemary, dried
- ½ teaspoon nutmeg, ground
- 1 and ½ cups veggie stock
- 1 tablespoon chives, chopped

Directions:
1. Grease the slow cooker with the oil, add the meat, onion, garlic and the other ingredients, toss, put the lid on and cook on Low for 7 hours.
2. Divide into bowls and serve for lunch.

Nutrition: calories 345, fat 7, fiber 5, carbs 14, protein 32

Turkey Chili

Preparation time: 10 minutes
Cooking time: 4 hours
Servings: 8

Ingredients:
- 1 red bell pepper, chopped
- 2 pounds turkey meat, ground
- 28 ounces canned tomatoes, chopped
- 1 red onion, chopped
- 1 green bell pepper, chopped
- 4 tablespoons tomato paste
- 1 tablespoon oregano, dried
- 3 tablespoon chili powder
- 3 tablespoons cumin, ground
- Salt and black pepper to the taste

Directions:
1. Heat up a pan over medium-high heat, add turkey, brown it for a few minutes, transfer to your slow cooker, add red and green bell pepper, onion, tomatoes, tomato paste, chili powder, oregano, cumin, salt and black pepper to the taste, stir, cover and cook on High for 4 hours.
2. Divide into bowls and serve for lunch.

Nutrition: calories 225, fat 6, fiber 4, carbs 15, protein 18

Pork and Tomatoes Mix

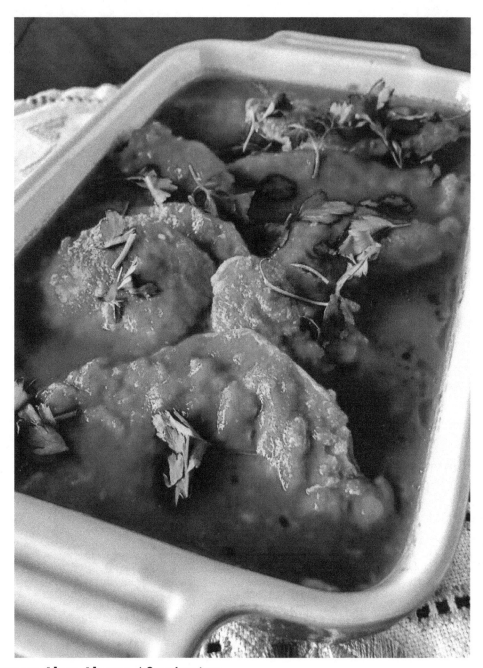

Preparation time: 10 minutes
Cooking time: 8 hours
Servings: 2

Ingredients:
- 1 and ½ pounds pork stew meat, cubed
- 1 cup cherry tomatoes, halved

- 1 cup tomato paste
- 1 tablespoon rosemary, chopped
- ½ teaspoon sweet paprika
- ½ teaspoon coriander, ground
- A pinch of salt and black pepper
- 1 tablespoon chives, chopped

Directions:

1. In your Crockpot, combine the meat with the tomatoes, tomato paste and the other ingredients, toss, put the lid on and cook on Low for 8 hours.
2. Divide between plates and serve for lunch.

Nutrition: calories 352, fat 8, fiber 4, carbs 10, protein 27

Turkey and Potatoes

Preparation time: 10 minutes
Cooking time: 8 hours
Servings: 4

Ingredients:
- 3 pounds turkey breast, skinless and boneless
- 1 cup cranberries, chopped
- 2 sweet potatoes, chopped
- ½ cup raisins
- ½ cup walnuts, chopped
- 1 sweet onion, chopped
- 2 tablespoons lemon juice
- 1 cup sugar
- 1 teaspoon ginger, grated
- ½ teaspoon nutmeg, ground
- 1 teaspoon cinnamon powder
- ½ cup veggie stock
- 1 teaspoon poultry seasoning
- Salt and black pepper to the taste
- 3 tablespoons olive oil

Directions:
1. Heat up a pan with the oil over medium-high heat, add cranberries, walnuts, raisins, onion, lemon juice, sugar, ginger, nutmeg, cinnamon, stock and black pepper, stir well and bring to a simmer.
2. Place turkey breast in your slow cooker, add sweet potatoes, cranberries mix and poultry seasoning, cover and cook on Low for 8 hours.
3. Slice turkey breast and divide between plates, add sweet potatoes, drizzle sauce from the slow cooker and serve for lunch.

Nutrition: calories 264, fat 4, fiber 6, carbs 8, protein 15

Pesto Pork Shanks

Preparation time: 10 minutes
Cooking time: 7 hours
Servings: 2

Ingredients:
- 1 and ½ pounds pork shanks
- 1 tablespoon olive oil
- 2 tablespoons basil pesto
- 1 red onion, sliced
- 1 cup beef stock
- ½ cup tomato paste
- 4 garlic cloves, minced
- 1 tablespoon oregano, chopped
- Zest and juice of 1 lemon
- A pinch of salt and black pepper

Directions:
1. In your slow cooker, mix the pork shanks with the oil, pesto and the other ingredients, toss, put the lid on and cook on Low for 7 hours.
2. Divide everything between plates and serve for lunch.

Nutrition: calories 372, fat 7, fiber 5, carbs 12, protein 37

Chicken Thighs Mix

Preparation time: 10 minutes
Cooking time: 6 hours
Servings: 6

Ingredients:
- 2 and ½ pounds chicken thighs, skinless and boneless
- 1 and ½ tablespoon olive oil
- 2 yellow onions, chopped
- 1 teaspoon cinnamon powder
- ¼ teaspoon cloves, ground
- ¼ teaspoon allspice, ground
- Salt and black pepper to the taste
- A pinch of saffron
- A handful pine nuts
- A handful mint, chopped

Directions:
1. In a bowl, mix oil with onions, cinnamon, allspice, cloves, salt, pepper and saffron, whisk and transfer to your slow cooker.
2. Add the chicken, toss well, cover and cook on Low for 6 hours.
3. Sprinkle pine nuts and mint on top before serving,

Nutrition: calories 223, fat 3, fiber 2, carbs 6, protein 13

Potato Stew

Preparation time: 10 minutes
Cooking time: 5 hours and 5 minutes
Servings: 4

Ingredients:

- ½ tablespoon olive oil
- 1 pound gold potatoes, peeled and cut into wedges
- 1 red onion, sliced
- 1 cup tomato paste
- ½ cup beef stock
- 1 carrot, sliced
- 1 red bell pepper, cubed
- 4 garlic cloves, minced
- 1 teaspoon sweet paprika
- 1 tablespoon chives, chopped

Directions:

1. Heat up a pan with the oil over medium-high heat, add the onion and garlic, sauté for 5 minutes and transfer to the slow cooker.
2. Add the potatoes and the other ingredients, toss, put the lid on and cook on Low for 5 hours.
3. Divide the stew into bowls and serve for lunch.

Nutrition: calories 273, fat 6, fiber 7, carbs 10, protein 17

Chicken and Stew

Preparation time: 10 minutes
Cooking time: 5 hours
Servings: 4

Ingredients:
- 4 chicken breasts, skinless and boneless
- 6 Italian sausages, sliced
- 5 garlic cloves, minced
- 1 white onion, chopped
- 1 teaspoon Italian seasoning
- A drizzle of olive oil
- 1 teaspoon garlic powder
- 29 ounces canned tomatoes, chopped
- 15 ounces tomato sauce
- 1 cup water
- ½ cup balsamic vinegar

Directions:
1. Put chicken and sausage slices in your slow cooker, add garlic, onion, Italian seasoning, oil, tomatoes, tomato sauce, garlic powder, water and the vinegar, cover and cook on High for 5 hours.
2. Stir the stew, divide between plates and serve for lunch

Nutrition: calories 267, fat 4, fiber 3, carbs 15, protein 13

Chicken and Rice

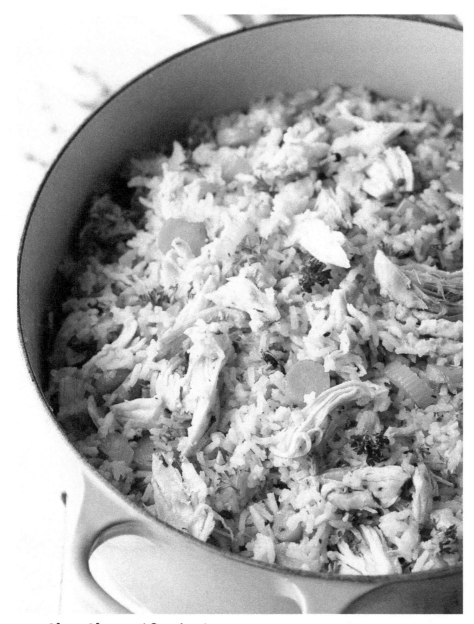

Preparation time: 10 minutes
Cooking time: 6 hours
Servings: 2

Ingredients:

- 1 pound chicken breast, skinless, boneless and cubed
- 1 red onion, sliced
- 2 spring onions, chopped

- Cooking spray
- 1 cup wild rice
- 2 cups chicken stock
- ½ teaspoon garam masala
- ½ teaspoon turmeric powder
- 1 tablespoon cilantro, chopped
- A pinch of salt and black pepper

Directions:

1. Grease the slow cooker with the cooking spray, add the chicken, rice, onion and the other ingredients, toss, put the lid on and cook on Low for 6 hours.
2. Divide the mix into bowls and serve for lunch.

Nutrition: calories 362, fat 8, fiber 8, carbs 10, protein 26

Chicken and Cabbage Mix

Preparation time: 10 minutes
Cooking time: 5 hours and 20 minutes
Servings: 6

Ingredients:
- 6 garlic cloves, minced
- 4 scallions, sliced
- 1 cup veggie stock
- 1 tablespoon olive oil
- 2 teaspoons sugar
- 1 tablespoon soy sauce
- 1 teaspoon ginger, minced
- 2 pounds chicken thighs, skinless and boneless
- 2 cups cabbage, shredded

Directions:
1. In your Slow cooker, mix stock with oil, scallions, garlic, sugar, soy sauce, ginger and chicken, stir, cover and cook on Low for 5 hours.
2. Transfer chicken to plates, add cabbage to the slow cooker, cover, cook on High for 20 minutes more, add next to the chicken and serve for lunch.

Nutrition: calories 240, fat 3, fiber 4, carbs 14, protein 10

Salmon Stew

Preparation time: 10 minutes
Cooking time: 2 hours
Servings: 4

Ingredients:
- 1 pound salmon fillets, boneless and roughly cubed
- 1 cup chicken stock
- ½ cup tomato paste
- ½ red onion, sliced
- 1 carrot, sliced
- 1 sweet potato, peeled and cubed
- 1 tablespoon cilantro, chopped
- Cooking spray
- ½ cup mild salsa
- 2 garlic cloves, minced
- A pinch of salt and black pepper

Directions:
1. In your slow cooker, mix the fish with the stock, tomato paste, onion and the other ingredients, toss gently, put the lid on and cook on Low for 2 hours
2. Divide the mix into bowls and serve for lunch.

Nutrition: calories 292, fat 6, fiber 7, carbs 12, protein 22

Pork and Chorizo Lunch Mix

Preparation time: 10 minutes
Cooking time: 4 hours
Servings: 8

Ingredients:
- 1 pound chorizo, ground
- 1 pound pork, ground
- 3 tablespoons olive oil
- 1 tomato, chopped
- 1 avocado, pitted, peeled and chopped
- Salt and black pepper to the taste
- 1 small red onion, chopped
- 2 tablespoons enchilada sauce

Directions:
1. Heat up a pan with the oil over medium-high heat, add pork, stir, brown for a couple of minutes, transfer to your slow cooker, add salt, pepper, chorizo, onion and enchilada sauce, stir, cover and cook on Low for 4 hours.
2. Divide between plates and serve with chopped tomato and avocado on top.

Nutrition: calories 300, fat 12, fiber 3, carbs 15, protein 17

Paprika Pork and Chickpeas

Preparation time: 10 minutes
Cooking time: 10 hours
Servings: 2

Ingredients:
- 1 red onion, sliced
- 1 pound pork stew meat, cubed
- 1 cup canned chickpeas, drained
- 1 cup beef stock
- 1 cup tomato paste
- ½ teaspoon sweet paprika
- ½ teaspoon turmeric powder
- A pinch of salt and black pepper
- 1 tablespoon hives, chopped

Directions:
1. In your slow cooker, mix the onion with the meat, chickpeas, stock and the other ingredients, toss, put the lid on and cook on Low for 10 hours.
2. Divide the mix between plates and serve for lunch.

Nutrition: calories 322, fat 6, fiber 6, carbs 9, protein 22

Lamb Stew

Preparation time: 10 minutes
Cooking time: 8 hours
Servings: 4

Ingredients:
- 1 and ½ pounds lamb meat, cubed
- ¼ cup flour
- Salt and black pepper to the taste
- 2 tablespoons olive oil
- 1 teaspoon rosemary, dried
- 1 onion, sliced
- ½ teaspoon thyme, dried
- 2 cups water
- 1 cup baby carrots
- 2 cups sweet potatoes, chopped

Directions:
1. In a bowl, mix lamb with flour and toss.
2. Heat up a pan with the oil over medium-high heat, add meat, brown it on all sides and transfer to your slow cooker.
3. Add onion, salt, pepper, rosemary, thyme, water, carrots and sweet potatoes, cover and cook on Low for 8 hours.
4. Divide lamb stew between plates and serve for lunch

Nutrition: calories 350, fat 8, fiber 3, carbs 20, protein 16

Beef and Cabbage

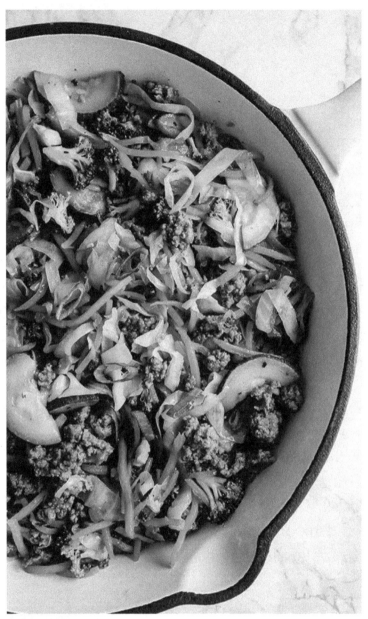

Preparation time: 10 minutes
Cooking time: 8 hours
Servings: 2

Ingredients:

- 1 pound beef stew meat, cubed
- 1 cup green cabbage, shredded
- 1 cup red cabbage, shredded

- 1 carrot, grated
- ½ cup water
- 1 cup tomato paste
- ½ teaspoon sweet paprika
- 1 tablespoon chives, chopped
- A pinch of salt and black pepper

Directions:
1. In your slow cooker, mix the beef with the cabbage, carrot and the other ingredients, toss, put the lid on and cook on Low for 8 hours.
2. Divide the mix between plates and serve for lunch.

Nutrition: calories 251, fat 6, fiber 7, carbs 12, protein 6

Lamb Curry

Preparation time: 10 minutes
Cooking time: 4 hours
Servings: 4

Ingredients:
- 1 and ½ tablespoons sweet paprika
- 3 tablespoons curry powder
- Salt and black pepper to the taste
- 2 pounds lamb meat, cubed
- 2 tablespoons olive oil
- 3 carrots, chopped
- 4 celery stalks, chopped
- 1 onion, chopped
- 4 celery stalks, chopped
- 1 cup chicken stock
- 4 garlic cloves minced
- 1 cup coconut milk

Directions:
1. Heat up a pan with the oil over medium-high heat, add lamb meat, brown it on all sides and transfer to your slow cooker.
2. Add stock, onions, celery and carrots to the slow cooker and stir everything gently.
3. In a bowl, mix paprika with a pinch of salt, black pepper and curry powder and stir.
4. Add spice mix to the cooker, also add coconut milk, cover, cook on High for 4 hours, divide into bowls and serve for lunch.

Nutrition: calories 300, fat 4, fiber 4, carbs 16, protein 13

Balsamic Beef Stew

Preparation time: 10 minutes
Cooking time: 6 hours
Servings: 2

Ingredients:
- 1 pound beef stew meat, cubed
- 1 teaspoon sweet paprika
- 1 red onion, sliced
- ½ cup mushrooms, sliced
- 1 carrot, peeled and cubed
- ½ cup tomatoes, cubed
- 1 tablespoon balsamic vinegar
- A pinch of salt and black pepper
- 1 teaspoon onion powder
- 1 teaspoon thyme, dried
- 1 cup beef stock
- 1 tablespoon cilantro, chopped

Directions:
1. In your slow cooker, mix the beef with the paprika, onion, mushrooms and the other ingredients except the cilantro, toss, put the lid on and cook on Low for 6 hours.
2. Divide into bowls and serve with the cilantro, sprinkled on top.

Nutrition: calories 322, fat 5, fiber 7, carbs 9, protein 16

Lamb and Bacon Stew

Preparation time: 10 minutes
Cooking time: 7 hours and 10 minutes
Servings: 6

Ingredients:
- 2 tablespoons flour
- 2 ounces bacon, cooked and crumbled
- 1 and ½ pounds lamb loin, chopped
- Salt and black pepper to the taste
- 1 garlic clove, minced
- 1 cup yellow onion, chopped
- 3 and ½ cups veggie stock
- 1 cup carrots, chopped
- 1 cup celery, chopped
- 2 cups sweet potatoes, chopped
- 1 tablespoon thyme, chopped
- 1 bay leaf
- 2 tablespoons olive oil

Directions:
1. Put lamb meat in a bowl, add flour, salt and pepper and toss to coat.
2. Heat up a pan with the oil over medium-high heat, add lamb, brown for 5 minutes on each side and transfer to your slow cooker.
3. Add onion, garlic, bacon, carrots, potatoes, bay leaf, stock, thyme and celery to the slow cooker as well, stir gently, cover and cook on Low for 7 hours.
4. Discard bay leaf, stir your stew, divide into bowls and serve for lunch

Nutrition: calories 360, fat 5, fiber 3, carbs 16, protein 17

Beef Curry

Preparation time: 10 minutes
Cooking time: 6 hours
Servings: 2

Ingredients:
- 1 pound beef stew meat
- 4 garlic cloves, minced
- 1 red onion, sliced
- 2 carrots, grated
- 1 tablespoon ginger, grated
- 2 tablespoons yellow curry paste
- 2 cups coconut milk
- A pinch of salt and black pepper

Directions:
1. In your slow cooker, mix the beef with the garlic, onion and the other ingredients, toss, put the lid on and cook on Low for 6 hours.
2. Divide the curry into bowls and serve for lunch.

Nutrition: calories 352, fat 6, fiber 7, carbs 9, protein 18

Sweet Potato Soup

Preparation time: 10 minutes
Cooking time: 5 hours and 20 minutes
Servings: 6

Ingredients:
- 5 cups veggie stock
- 3 sweet potatoes, peeled and chopped
- 2 celery stalks, chopped
- 1 cup yellow onion, chopped
- 1 cup milk
- 1 teaspoon tarragon, dried
- 2 garlic cloves, minced
- 2 cups baby spinach
- 8 tablespoons almonds, sliced
- Salt and black pepper to the taste

Directions:
1. In your slow cooker, mix stock with potatoes, celery, onion, milk, tarragon, garlic, salt and pepper, stir, cover and cook on High for 5 hours.
2. Blend soup using an immersion blender, add spinach and almonds, toss, cover and leave aside for 20 minutes.
3. Divide soup into bowls and serve for lunch.

Nutrition: calories 301, fat 5, fiber 4, carbs 12, protein 5

Chicken and Brussels Sprouts Mix

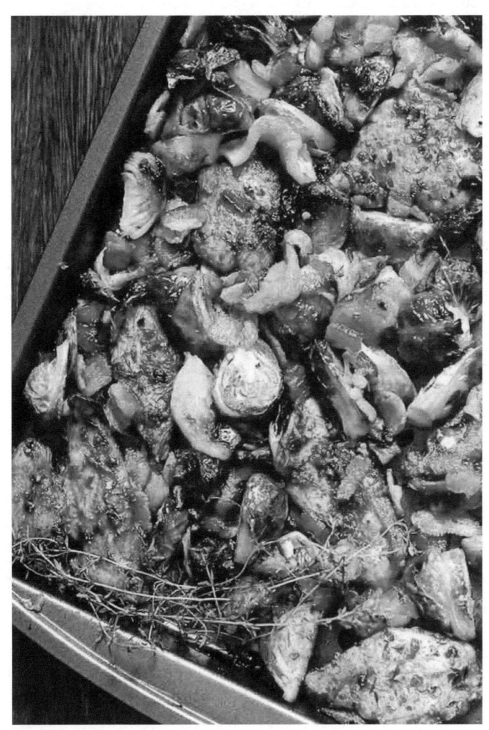

Preparation time: 10 minutes
Cooking time: 6 hours
Servings: 2

Ingredients:

- 1 pound chicken breast, skinless, boneless and cubed
- 1 red onion, sliced
- 1 cup Brussels sprouts, trimmed and halved
- 1 cup chicken stock
- ½ cup tomato paste
- A pinch of salt and black pepper
- 1 garlic clove, crushed
- 1 tablespoon thyme, chopped
- 1 tablespoon rosemary, chopped

Directions:

1. In your slow cooker, mix the chicken with the onion, sprouts and the other ingredients, toss, put the lid on and cook on Low for 6 hours.
2. Divide the mix between plates and serve for lunch.

Nutrition: calories 261, fat 7, fiber 6, carbs 8, protein 26

White Beans Stew

Preparation time: 10 minutes
Cooking time: 4 hours
Servings: 10

Ingredients:
- 2 pounds white beans
- 3 celery stalks, chopped
- 2 carrots, chopped
- 1 bay leaf
- 1 yellow onion, chopped
- 3 garlic cloves, minced
- 1 teaspoon rosemary, dried
- 1 teaspoon oregano, dried
- 1 teaspoon thyme, dried
- 10 cups water
- Salt and black pepper to the taste
- 28 ounces canned tomatoes, chopped
- 6 cups chard, chopped

Directions:
1. In your slow cooker, mix white beans with celery, carrots, bay leaf, onion, garlic, rosemary, oregano, thyme, water, salt, pepper, tomatoes and chard, cover and cook on High for 4 hours.
2. Stir, divide into bowls and serve for lunch,

Nutrition: calories 341, fat 8, fiber 12, carbs 20, protein 6

Chickpeas Stew

Preparation time: 10 minutes
Cooking time: 3 hours
Servings: 4

Ingredients:
- 2 cups canned chickpeas, drained and rinsed
- 1 cup tomato sauce
- ½ cup chicken stock
- 1 red onion, sliced
- 2 garlic cloves, minced
- 1 tablespoon thyme, chopped
- ½ teaspoon turmeric powder
- ½ teaspoon garam masala
- 2 carrots, chopped
- 3 celery stalks, chopped
- 2 tablespoons parsley, chopped
- A pinch of salt and black pepper

Directions:
1. In your slow cooker, mix the chickpeas with the tomato sauce, chicken stock and the other ingredients, toss, put the lid on and cook on High for 3 hours.
2. Divide into bowls and serve for lunch.

Nutrition: calories 300, fat 4, fiber 7, carbs 9, protein 22

Bulgur Chili

Preparation time: 10 minutes
Cooking time: 8 hours
Servings: 4

Ingredients:
- 2 cups white mushrooms, sliced
- ¾ cup bulgur, soaked in 1 cup hot water for 15 minutes and drained
- 2 cups yellow onion, chopped
- ½ cup red bell pepper, chopped
- 1 cup veggie stock
- 2 garlic cloves, minced
- 1 cup strong brewed coffee
- 14 ounces canned kidney beans, drained
- 14 ounces canned pinto beans, drained
- 2 tablespoons sugar
- 2 tablespoons chili powder
- 1 tablespoon cocoa powder
- 1 teaspoon oregano, dried
- 2 teaspoons cumin, ground
- 1 bay leaf
- Salt and black pepper to the taste

Directions:
1. In your Slow cooker, mix mushrooms with bulgur, onion, bell pepper, stock, garlic, coffee, kidney and pinto beans, sugar, chili powder, cocoa, oregano, cumin, bay leaf, salt and pepper, stir gently, cover and cook on Low for 12 hours.
2. Discard bay leaf, divide chili into bowls and serve for lunch.

Nutrition: calories 351, fat 4, fiber 6, carbs 20, protein 4

Eggplant Curry

Preparation time: 10 minutes
Cooking time: 3 hours
Servings: 2

Ingredients:
- 2 tablespoons olive oil
- 1 pound eggplant, cubed
- 2 tablespoons red curry paste
- 1 cup coconut milk
- ½ cup veggie stock
- 1 teaspoon turmeric powder
- ½ teaspoon rosemary, dried
- 4 kaffir lime leaves

Directions:
1. In your slow cooker, mix the eggplant with the oil, curry paste and the other ingredients, toss, put the lid on and cook on High for 3 hours.
2. Discard lime leaves, divide the curry into bowls and serve for lunch.

Nutrition: calories 281, fat 7, fiber 6, carbs 8, protein 22

Quinoa Chili

Preparation time: 10 minutes
Cooking time: 6 hours
Servings: 6

Ingredients:
- 2 cups veggie stock
- ½ cup quinoa
- 30 ounces canned black beans, drained
- 28 ounces canned tomatoes, chopped
- 1 green bell pepper, chopped
- 1 yellow onion, chopped
- 2 sweet potatoes, cubed
- 1 tablespoon chili powder
- 2 tablespoons cocoa powder
- 2 teaspoons cumin, ground
- Salt and black pepper to the taste
- ¼ teaspoon smoked paprika

Directions:
1. In your slow cooker, mix stock with quinoa, black beans, tomatoes, bell pepper, onion, sweet potatoes, chili powder, cocoa, cumin, paprika, salt and pepper, stir, cover and cook on High for 6 hours.
2. Divide into bowls and serve for lunch.

Nutrition: calories 342, fat 6, fiber 7, carbs 18, protein 4

Beef and Artichokes Stew

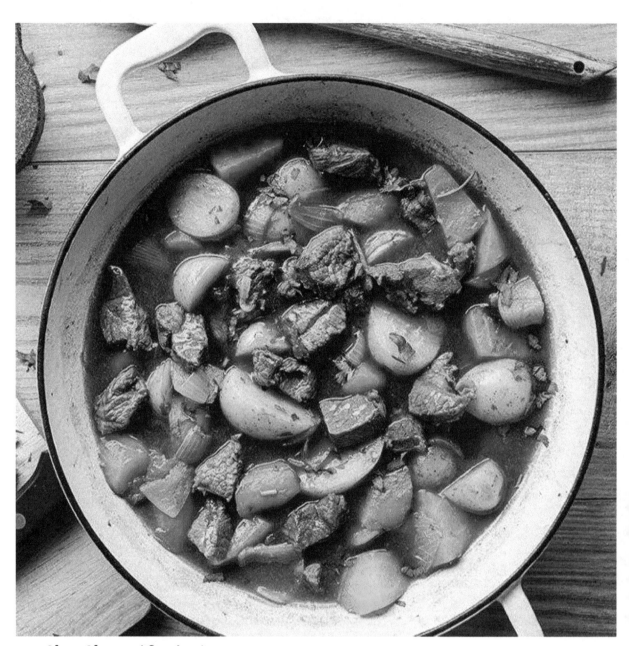

Preparation time: 10 minutes
Cooking time: 4 hours
Servings: 2

Ingredients:

- 1 pound beef stew meat, cubed
- 1 cup canned artichoke hearts, halved
- 1 cup beef stock

- 1 red onion, sliced
- 1 cup tomato sauce
- ½ teaspoon rosemary, dried
- ½ teaspoon coriander, ground
- 1 teaspoon garlic powder
- A drizzle of olive oil
- A pinch of salt and black pepper
- 1 tablespoon chives, chopped

Directions:
1. Grease the slow cooker with the oil and mix the beef with the artichokes, stock and the other ingredients inside.
2. Toss, put the lid on and cook on High for 4 hours.
3. Divide the stew into bowls and serve.

Nutrition: calories 322, fat 5, fiber 4, carbs 12, protein 22

Pumpkin Chili

Preparation time: 10 minutes
Cooking time: 5 hours
Servings: 6

Ingredients:
- 1 cup pumpkin puree
- 30 ounces canned kidney beans, drained
- 30 ounces canned roasted tomatoes, chopped
- 2 cups water
- 1 cup red lentils, dried
- 1 cup yellow onion, chopped
- 1 jalapeno pepper, chopped
- 1 tablespoon chili powder
- 1 tablespoon cocoa powder
- ½ teaspoon cinnamon powder
- 2 teaspoons cumin, ground
- A pinch of cloves, ground
- Salt and black pepper to the taste
- 2 tomatoes, chopped

Directions:
1. In your Slow cooker, mix pumpkin puree with kidney beans, roasted tomatoes, water, lentils, onion, jalapeno, chili powder, cocoa, cinnamon, cumin, cloves, salt and pepper, stir, cover and cook on High for 5 hours.
2. Divide into bowls, top with chopped tomatoes and serve for lunch.

Nutrition: calories 266, fat 6, fiber 4, carbs 12, protein 4

Beef Soup

Preparation time: 10 minutes
Cooking time: 5 hours
Servings: 2

Ingredients:
- 1 pound beef stew meat, cubed
- 3 cups beef stock
- ½ cup tomatoes, cubed
- 1 red onion, chopped
- 1 green bell pepper, chopped
- 1 carrot, cubed
- A pinch of salt and black pepper
- ½ tablespoon oregano, dried
- ¼ teaspoon chili pepper
- 2 tablespoon tomato paste
- 1 jalapeno, chopped
- 1 tablespoon cilantro, chopped

Directions:
1. In your slow cooker, mix the beef with the stock, tomatoes and the other ingredients, toss, put the lid on and cook on Low for 5 hours.
2. Divide the soup into bowls and serve for lunch.

Nutrition: calories 391, fat 6, fiber 7, carbs 8, protein 27

3 Bean Chili

Preparation time: 10 minutes
Cooking time: 8 hours
Servings: 6

Ingredients:
- 15 ounces canned kidney beans, drained
- 30 ounces canned chili beans in sauce
- 15 ounces canned black beans, drained
- 2 green bell peppers, chopped
- 30 ounces canned tomatoes, crushed
- 2 tablespoons chili powder
- 2 yellow onions, chopped
- 2 garlic cloves, minced
- 1 teaspoon oregano, dried
- 1 tablespoon cumin, ground
- Salt and black pepper to the taste

Directions:
1. In your Slow cooker, mix kidney beans with chili beans, black beans, bell peppers, tomatoes, chili powder, onion, garlic, oregano, cumin, salt and pepper, stir, cover and cook on Low for 8 hours.
2. Divide into bowls and serve for lunch.

Nutrition: calories 314, fat 6, fiber 5, carbs 14, protein 4

Conclusion

Did you delight in attempting these new and delicious dishes? regrettably we have actually come to the end of this vegetarian recipe book, I actually hope it has actually been to your taste. to improve your health and wellness we want to encourage you to combine physical activity as well as a dynamic way of life as well as adhere to these amazing dishes, so regarding emphasize the enhancements. we will certainly be back soon with various other significantly fascinating vegan dishes, a big hug, see you quickly.

CPSIA information can be obtained
at www.ICGtesting.com
Printed in the USA
LVHW060902290521
688445LV00038B/975